MEDITERRANEAN DIET COOKBOOK FOR RHEUMATOID ARTHRITIS

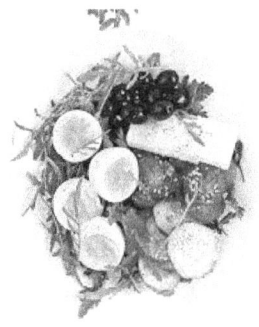

30 Essential anti-inflammatory recipes to fight arthritis, fatigue, and inflammation

Dr. Mary D. Cook

OTHER BOOKS BY THE AUTHOR

1. OSTEOPOROSIS DIET COOKBOOK FOR SENIORS

CLICK HERE TO GET YOUR COPY NOW!!!

2. THE ULTIMATE GASTRIC SLEEVE BARIATRIC COOKBOOK

CLICK HERE TO GET YOUR COPY!!!

3. PESCATARIAN DIET COOKBOOK FOR DIABETICS

CLICK HER TO GET YOUR COPY NOW!!!

TABLE OF CONTENTS

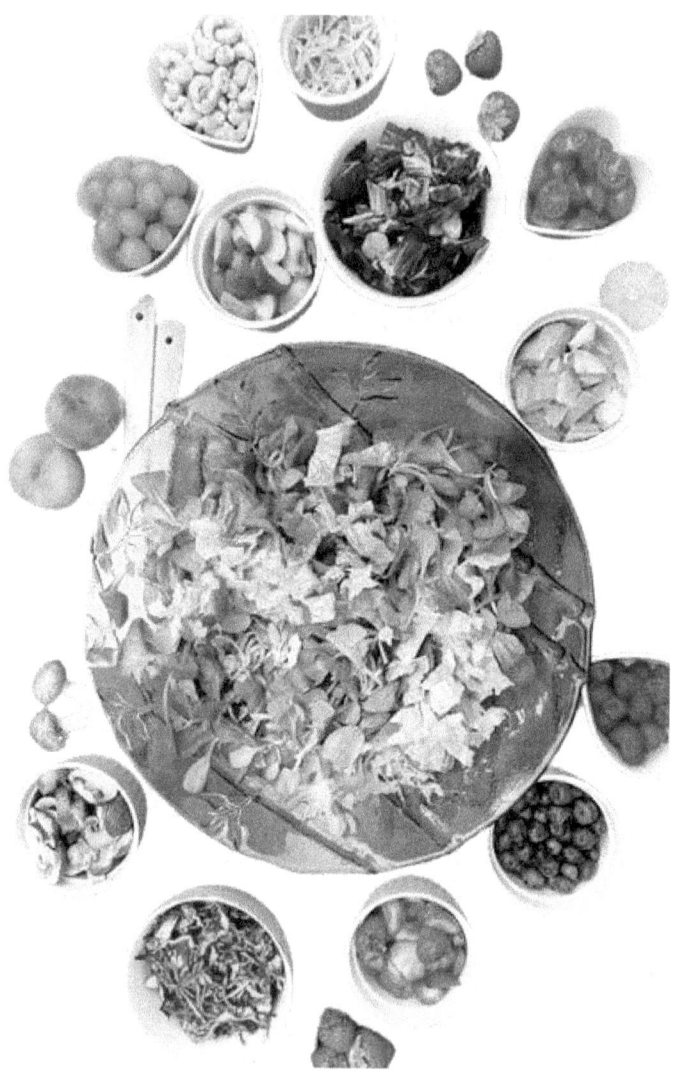

INTRODUCTION

Welcome to a culinary journey designed not just to tantalize your taste buds but to nourish your body and soul. I'm Dr. Mary D. Cook, a seasoned nutritionist, and it is my pleasure to guide you through a transformative experience with the **"Mediterranean Diet Cookbook for Rheumatoid Arthritis."** In these pages, we embark on a quest to harness the healing power of food, embracing a diet that not only delights the senses but also becomes a potent ally in your battle against rheumatoid arthritis.

Living with rheumatoid arthritis is a unique challenge that extends beyond the physical realm. It's a journey of resilience, strength, and a steadfast commitment to one's well-being. Having witnessed the impact of nutrition on health throughout my career, I felt compelled to create a cookbook tailored to those navigating the complexities of rheumatoid arthritis. The Mediterranean diet, renowned for its holistic benefits, emerged as the perfect cornerstone for this culinary endeavor.

Years ago, my sister Linda faced the daunting challenge of rheumatoid arthritis, a relentless adversary that sought to compromise her quality of life. Witnessing her pain and discomfort, I knew that conventional approaches were not enough. It was a pivotal moment that fueled my determination to explore the profound impact of nutrition on health.

In our pursuit of a solution, I embarked on a mission to harness the healing potential of the Mediterranean diet, renowned for its anti-inflammatory properties and its ability to promote overall well-being. The journey wasn't easy, but with dedication and a commitment to embracing a lifestyle centered around nutritious, flavorful meals, Linda experienced a remarkable transformation.

Through the pages of this cookbook, I share not only the recipes that played a pivotal role in Linda's recovery but also the knowledge that can empower you to take charge of your health. Linda's story is a testament to the fact that food is not just sustenance; it is medicine. Together, we can embark on a journey to harness the healing power of nutrition, just as Linda did.

CHAPTER: 1

Rheumatoid Arthritis:

Rheumatoid Arthritis (RA) stands as a formidable adversary within the realm of autoimmune diseases, affecting millions of individuals worldwide. This chronic inflammatory disorder not only impacts the joints but also poses significant challenges to overall health and well-being. To comprehend the intricate nature of RA, one must delve into its types, causes, symptoms, and preventive measures.

Understanding Rheumatoid Arthritis:

Rheumatoid Arthritis is a chronic autoimmune disorder characterized by inflammation primarily affecting the synovium, the lining of the membranes that surround the joints. Unlike osteoarthritis, which is more common and results from wear and tear on the joints, RA involves the immune system mistakenly attacking the body's own tissues.

Types of Rheumatoid Arthritis:

While RA often presents itself in a similar manner, there are variations in its manifestation that warrant recognition. Seropositive RA is marked by the presence of specific antibodies, such as rheumatoid factor (RF) and anti-citrullinated protein antibodies (ACPAs), in the blood. Seronegative RA, on the other hand, lacks these markers, posing diagnostic challenges. Additionally, juvenile idiopathic arthritis (JIA) is a subtype affecting children, further highlighting the diverse nature of this condition.

Causes of Rheumatoid Arthritis:

The exact cause of RA remains elusive, but it is widely accepted that a combination of genetic and environmental factors contributes to its development. Genetic predisposition is a significant factor, with certain genes, such as the HLA-DRB1 gene, being associated with an increased susceptibility to RA. Environmental triggers, including infections and exposure to certain pollutants, may act as catalysts, initiating the autoimmune response in genetically predisposed individuals.

Symptoms of Rheumatoid Arthritis:

RA's onset is often insidious, with symptoms gradually intensifying over time. Joint pain, swelling, and stiffness are hallmark features, typically affecting smaller joints first, such as those in the hands and feet. Morning stiffness, lasting for more than an hour, is a common complaint. As the disease progresses, larger joints may become involved, and systemic symptoms such as fatigue, weight loss, and a general feeling of malaise may accompany joint-related issues.

Preventive Measures for Rheumatoid Arthritis:

While there is no foolproof method to prevent RA, adopting a proactive and health-conscious lifestyle can significantly reduce the risk or help manage the condition effectively.

Maintain a Healthy Lifestyle: Regular exercise is crucial in promoting joint health and flexibility. Low-impact activities such as swimming, walking, and yoga can be particularly beneficial.

A balanced diet rich in antioxidants, omega-3 fatty acids, and other anti-inflammatory nutrients supports overall health.

Early Diagnosis and Treatment: Timely identification of RA is paramount. Early intervention with disease-modifying antirheumatic drugs (DMARDs) can slow down the progression of the disease, preventing irreversible joint damage.

Manage Stress: Stress has been implicated in triggering RA flares. Incorporating stress management techniques such as meditation, deep breathing exercises, and mindfulness into daily life can contribute to overall well-being.

Regular Health Check-ups: Regular visits to healthcare professionals for check-ups and monitoring are essential, especially for individuals with a family history of RA or those displaying early symptoms.

Avoid Smoking: Smoking has been identified as a significant environmental risk factor for developing RA. Quitting smoking can not only reduce the risk of RA but also improve the overall health of individuals.

Navigating the Journey with Knowledge and Empowerment

In the realm of autoimmune diseases, Rheumatoid Arthritis poses a formidable challenge, demanding a comprehensive understanding of its nuances for effective management. From recognizing its diverse types to unraveling the intricate web of causes and symptoms, and finally, embracing preventive measures, knowledge emerges as a powerful tool in navigating the complexities of RA.

While the path of Rheumatoid Arthritis may be daunting, there is hope in the proactive measures one can take. By fostering a lifestyle that nurtures joint health, seeking early diagnosis and treatment, and adopting strategies to manage stress, individuals can empower themselves in the face of this chronic condition. With ongoing research and a commitment to raising awareness, the journey towards a future with improved treatments and, eventually, a cure for Rheumatoid Arthritis continues.

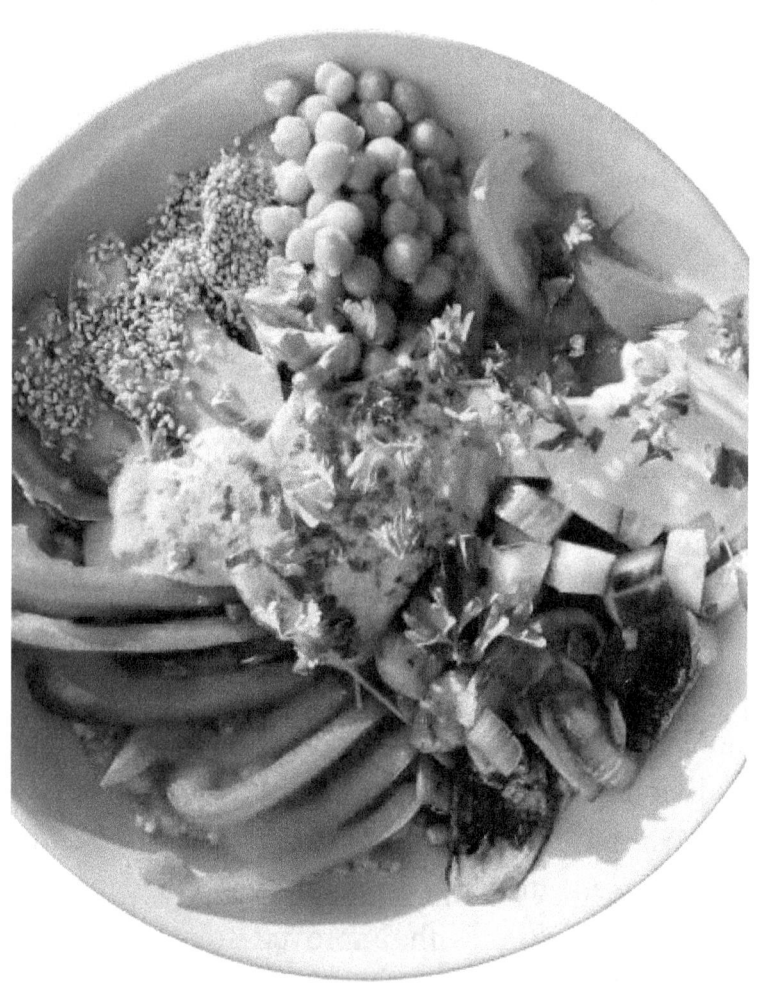

CHAPTER: 2

A Rheumatoid Arthritis Diet Guide:

Rheumatoid Arthritis (RA) is a chronic condition that not only affects joints but also influences overall health. While there's no singular "magic" diet to cure RA, adopting a well-balanced and thoughtful approach to nutrition can play a crucial role in managing symptoms and promoting overall well-being. Here's a guide on foods to include and avoid for those navigating the path of a Rheumatoid Arthritis diet.

Foods to Include:

Fatty Fish: Omega-3 fatty acids found in fish like salmon, mackerel, and sardines possess anti-inflammatory properties. Incorporating these into your diet can help manage inflammation associated with RA.

Colorful Fruits and Vegetables: Rich in antioxidants, vitamins, and minerals, fruits and vegetables contribute to overall health. Berries, cherries, broccoli, spinach, and sweet potatoes are particularly beneficial for their anti-inflammatory properties.

Whole Grains: Opt for whole grains like brown rice, quinoa, and oats. These grains provide fiber and essential nutrients, promoting gut health and aiding in weight management.

Nuts and Seeds: Almonds, walnuts, and flaxseeds are excellent sources of healthy fats, fiber, and antioxidants. They can be a valuable addition to your diet to support joint health.

Olive Oil: Extra virgin olive oil is a staple of the Mediterranean diet, known for its anti-inflammatory effects. It can be used in cooking or as a salad dressing.

Lean Proteins: Incorporate lean protein sources like poultry, tofu, and legumes. Protein is crucial for maintaining muscle mass and supporting the body's repair processes.

Dairy or Dairy Alternatives: Calcium is essential for bone health. Include dairy or fortified dairy alternatives to meet your calcium needs.

Spices: Turmeric and ginger have natural anti-inflammatory properties.

Consider adding these spices to your meals for both flavor and potential health benefits.

Foods to Avoid: Minimizing Triggers for Inflammation

1. **Processed Foods:** High in preservatives, additives, and unhealthy fats, processed foods can contribute to inflammation. Opt for fresh, whole foods instead.

2. **Saturated and Trans Fats:** Reducing intake of saturated fats found in red meat and full-fat dairy, as well as trans fats in processed and fried foods, may help manage inflammation.

3. **Refined Carbohydrates:** White bread, pasta, and sugary snacks can contribute to inflammation and may lead to weight gain. Choose whole grains and limit refined carbohydrates.

4. **Sugar and Artificial Sweeteners:** Excessive sugar intake can contribute to inflammation. Read labels and be mindful of hidden sugars. Artificial sweeteners may also have inflammatory effects in some individuals.

5. **Alcohol:** While moderate alcohol consumption may have some cardiovascular

benefits, excessive alcohol intake can exacerbate inflammation and interfere with medication effectiveness.

6. **Nightshade Vegetables:** Some individuals with RA find that nightshade vegetables like tomatoes, eggplants, and peppers may worsen symptoms. Pay attention to your body's response and consider limiting or avoiding these if needed.

7. **Excessive Salt:** High sodium intake can contribute to water retention and may exacerbate inflammation. Be mindful of salt content in processed foods and try to limit added salt in cooking.

Conclusion: Crafting a Personalized Approach

A Rheumatoid Arthritis diet is not one-size-fits-all. Individual responses to specific foods can vary, and it's crucial to listen to your body. Remember, a well-rounded approach to diet and lifestyle can contribute significantly to your overall well-being and quality of life.

Core benefits of following a Rheumatoid Arthritis diet

Adopting a Rheumatoid Arthritis (RA) diet can offer a range of benefits, contributing to better management of symptoms and an overall improvement in health. Here are some core benefits:

1. **Reduced Inflammation:** One of the primary goals of an RA diet is to minimize inflammation, a key driver of pain and joint damage in individuals with rheumatoid arthritis. Foods rich in omega-3 fatty acids, antioxidants, and anti-inflammatory properties can help in this regard.

2. **Joint Health and Mobility:** Certain nutrients, such as omega-3 fatty acids found in fatty fish, have been associated with improved joint health. By supporting joint function and reducing stiffness, an RA diet can contribute to enhanced mobility and a better quality of life.

3. **Weight Management:** Maintaining a healthy weight is crucial for individuals with RA. Excess weight puts additional strain on joints, exacerbating symptoms. A well-balanced diet that includes nutrient-dense foods helps in weight management, promoting joint health and reducing the impact of excess body weight.

4. **Support for Bone Health:** Some individuals with RA may be at a higher risk of osteoporosis due to factors such as inflammation and the use of certain medications. A diet rich in calcium and vitamin D, found in dairy products and fortified foods, supports bone health and helps mitigate the risk of fractures.

5. **Balanced Nutrition for Overall Well-Being:** The emphasis on whole, nutrient-dense foods in an RA diet ensures a well-rounded nutritional profile. Fruits, vegetables, lean proteins, and whole grains provide essential vitamins and minerals necessary for overall health, immune function, and energy levels.

6. **Improved Gut Health:** A healthy gut microbiome is increasingly recognized for its role in immune function and inflammation. Including fiber-rich foods, such as fruits, vegetables, and whole grains, supports a diverse and balanced gut microbiota, contributing to overall well-being.

7. **Optimized Medication Effectiveness:** Some nutrients can interact with medications, influencing their absorption or efficacy. A carefully planned diet, coordinated with healthcare professionals, ensures that the medications prescribed for managing RA are optimally effective.

8. **Enhanced Energy Levels:** Chronic conditions like RA can often lead to fatigue. A well-balanced diet that includes a mix of macronutrients (carbohydrates, proteins, and fats) and micronutrients provides the energy needed for daily activities, reducing fatigue and supporting a more active lifestyle.

9. **Joint Protection and Disease Progression:** By focusing on anti-inflammatory foods and avoiding potential triggers, an RA diet may help protect joints from further damage. Early intervention with a supportive diet can contribute to slowing the progression of the disease and preserving joint function.

10. **Improved Mood and Mental Well-Being:** Chronic conditions can take a toll on mental health. Nutrient-dense foods, including those rich in omega-3 fatty acids, have been associated with improved mood and cognitive function. A positive impact on mental well-being contributes to an overall better quality of life for individuals with RA.

It's important to note that individual responses to specific foods can vary, and there is no one-size-fits-all approach to an RA diet. Consulting with healthcare professionals, including a registered dietitian, can help tailor dietary recommendations to an individual's specific needs and preferences, maximizing the potential benefits of a rheumatoid arthritis-focused nutrition plan.

CHAPTER 3: BREAKFAST RECIPES

1. Greek Yogurt Parfait with Berries and Nuts

Ingredients:

- 1 cup Greek yogurt (unsweetened)
- 1/2 cup mixed berries (blueberries, strawberries)
- 2 tablespoons chopped almonds or walnuts
- 1 teaspoon honey (optional)

Instructions:

1. In a serving bowl, layer Greek yogurt.
2. Add a layer of mixed berries.
3. Sprinkle chopped nuts on top.
4. Drizzle with honey if desired.
5. Serve immediately.

Nutritional Value (per serving): Calories: 250, Protein: 20g, Fiber: 4g, Calcium: 200mg, Vitamin D: 5 IU

Cooking Time: 5 minutes

2. Mediterranean Avocado Toast with Tomatoes and Feta

Ingredients:

- 1 slice whole-grain bread
- 1/2 ripe avocado
- 1 medium tomato, sliced
- 1 tablespoon crumbled feta cheese
- Fresh basil leaves for garnish

Instructions:

1. Toast the whole-grain bread.
2. Mash the avocado and spread it on the toast.
3. Arrange tomato slices on top.
4. Sprinkle crumbled feta cheese.
5. Garnish with fresh basil leaves.
6. Serve immediately.

Nutritional Value (per serving): Calories: 280, Protein: 8g, Fiber: 7g, Calcium: 60mg, Vitamin D: 2 IU

Cooking Time: 10 minutes

3. Mediterranean Veggie Omelette

Ingredients:

- 2 large eggs
- 1/4 cup diced bell peppers (mixed colors)
- 1/4 cup cherry tomatoes, halved
- 2 tablespoons feta cheese, crumbled
- Fresh parsley for garnish
- Olive oil for cooking

Instructions:

1. Whisk eggs in a bowl.
2. Heat olive oil in a pan.
3. Sauté bell peppers and cherry tomatoes until soft.
4. Pour whisked eggs over veggies.
5. Once set, sprinkle feta cheese and fold the omelette.
6. Garnish with fresh parsley.
7. Serve hot.

Nutritional Value (per serving): Calories: 280, Protein: 18g, Fiber: 3g, Calcium: 150mg, Vitamin D: 4 IU

Cooking Time: 15 minutes

---

4. Quinoa Breakfast Bowl with Mediterranean Flavors

Ingredients:

- 1/2 cup cooked quinoa
- 1/4 cup cucumber, diced
- 1/4 cup cherry tomatoes, halved
- 2 tablespoons Kalamata olives, sliced
- 1 tablespoon feta cheese, crumbled
- Fresh mint leaves for garnish

Instructions:

1. In a bowl, mix cooked quinoa with diced cucumber.
2. Add cherry tomatoes and Kalamata olives.
3. Sprinkle crumbled feta cheese.

4. Garnish with fresh mint leaves.

5. Serve at room temperature.

Nutritional Value (per serving): Calories: 220, Protein: 8g, Fiber: 5g, Calcium: 100mg, Vitamin D: 3 IU

Cooking Time: 20 minutes

---

5. Mediterranean Chia Seed Pudding

Ingredients:

- 2 tablespoons chia seeds
- 1/2 cup unsweetened almond milk
- 1/4 cup Greek yogurt
- 1/2 teaspoon vanilla extract
- 1 tablespoon sliced almonds
- Fresh berries for topping

Instructions:

1. Mix chia seeds, almond milk, Greek yogurt, and vanilla extract in a jar.

2. Refrigerate overnight or for at least 4 hours.

3. Top with sliced almonds and fresh berries.

4. Serve chilled.

Nutritional Value (per serving): Calories: 180, Protein: 8g, Fiber: 10g, Calcium: 200mg, Vitamin D: 2 IU

Cooking/Prep Time: 5 minutes (plus refrigeration)

---

6. Spinach and Feta Stuffed Mushrooms

Ingredients:

- 4 large mushrooms, cleaned and stems removed
- 1 cup fresh spinach, chopped
- 2 tablespoons feta cheese, crumbled
- 1 clove garlic, minced
- Olive oil for drizzling

Instructions:

1. Preheat oven to 375°F (190°C).

2. In a bowl, mix chopped spinach, feta cheese, and minced garlic.

3. Stuff mushrooms with the spinach mixture.

4. Drizzle with olive oil.

5. Bake for 15-20 minutes or until mushrooms are tender. Serve warm.

Nutritional Value (per serving): Calories: 120, Protein: 7g, Fiber: 3g, Calcium: 80mg, Vitamin D: 1 IU

Cooking Time: 20 minutes

---

7. Mediterranean Tofu Scramble

Ingredients:

- 1/2 cup firm tofu, crumbled
- 1/4 cup cherry tomatoes, halved
- 2 tablespoons black olives, sliced
- 1 tablespoon nutritional yeast
- Fresh oregano for garnish
- Olive oil for cooking

Instructions:

1. Heat olive oil in a pan.

2. Add crumbled tofu and cook until slightly browned.

3. Stir in cherry tomatoes and black olives.

4. Sprinkle nutritional yeast over the mixture.

5. Cook until tomatoes are soft.

6. Garnish with fresh oregano.

7. Serve hot.

Nutritional Value (per serving):

- Calories: 220

- Protein: 15g

- Fiber: 4g

- Calcium: 200mg

- Vitamin D: 2 IU

Cooking Time: 15 minutes

8. Mediterranean Smoothie Bowl

Ingredients:

- 1/2 cup frozen mixed berries
- 1/2 banana, frozen
- 1/2 cup Greek yogurt
- 1 tablespoon chia seeds
- 1 tablespoon honey
- Sliced almonds for topping

Instructions:

1. Blend frozen berries, frozen banana, Greek yogurt, and chia seeds until smooth.
2. Pour into a bowl.
3. Drizzle honey on top.
4. Sprinkle sliced almonds.
5. Serve immediately.

Nutritional Value (per serving):

- Calories: 280

- Protein: 15g
- Fiber: 7g
- Calcium: 250mg
- Vitamin D: 3 IU

Prep Time: 5 minutes

---

9. Mediterranean Shakshuka

Ingredients:

- 2 eggs
- 1/2 cup tomato sauce (no added sugar)
- 1/4 cup bell peppers, diced
- 1/4 cup onion, diced
- 1 clove garlic, minced
- 1/2 teaspoon cumin
- Fresh cilantro for garnish

Instructions:

1. In a pan, sauté diced bell peppers, onions, and minced garlic.

2. Add tomato sauce and cumin, simmer for a few minutes.

3. Create wells in the sauce and crack eggs into them.

4. Cover and cook until eggs are done.

5. Garnish with fresh cilantro.

6. Serve hot.

Nutritional Value (per serving):

- Calories: 230
- Protein: 14g
- Fiber: 4g
- Calcium: 120mg
- Vitamin D: 3 IU

Cooking Time: 20 minutes

10. Mediterranean Overnight Oats

Ingredients:

- 1/2 cup rolled oats

- 1/2 cup unsweetened almond milk

- 1/4 cup plain Greek yogurt

- 1 tablespoon chia seeds

- 1/4 cup mixed fresh berries

- 1 tablespoon chopped pistachios

Instructions:

1. In a jar, combine rolled oats, almond milk, Greek yogurt, and chia seeds.

2. Mix well and refrigerate overnight.

3. In the morning, top with mixed fresh berries and chopped pistachios.

4. Serve chilled.

Nutritional Value (per serving): Calories: 270, Protein: 12g, Fiber: 8g, Calcium: 200mg, Vitamin D: 2 IU

Prep Time: 5 minutes (plus refrigeration)

CHAPTER 4: LUNCH RECIPES

1. Mediterranean Chickpea Salad

Ingredients:

- 1 can (15 oz) chickpeas, drained and rinsed
- 1 cup cherry tomatoes, halved
- 1 cucumber, diced
- 1/2 red onion, finely chopped
- 1/4 cup feta cheese, crumbled
- 2 tablespoons extra virgin olive oil
- 1 tablespoon lemon juice
- 1 teaspoon dried oregano
- Salt and pepper to taste
- Fresh parsley for garnish

Instructions:

1. In a large bowl, combine chickpeas, cherry tomatoes, cucumber, red onion, and feta cheese.

2. In a small bowl, whisk together olive oil, lemon juice, dried oregano, salt, and pepper.

3. Pour the dressing over the salad and toss to combine.

4. Garnish with fresh parsley.

5. Serve chilled.

Nutritional Value (per serving):

- Calories: 320

- Protein: 12g

- Fiber: 8g

- Calcium: 120mg

- Vitamin D: 2 IU

Cooking Time: 15 minutes

2. Mediterranean Grilled Chicken Skewers

Ingredients:

- 1 lb boneless, skinless chicken breast, cut into chunks
- 1 bell pepper, cut into chunks
- 1 zucchini, sliced
- 1 red onion, cut into wedges
- 2 tablespoons olive oil
- 1 teaspoon dried rosemary
- 1 teaspoon dried thyme
- Salt and pepper to taste
- Lemon wedges for serving

Instructions:

1. In a bowl, toss chicken, bell pepper, zucchini, and red onion with olive oil, rosemary, thyme, salt, and pepper.

2. Thread onto skewers.

3. Grill skewers over medium heat until chicken is cooked through, about 10-12 minutes.

4. Serve with lemon wedges.

Nutritional Value (per serving): Calories: 280, Protein: 30g, Fiber: 4g, Calcium: 40mg, Vitamin D: 2 IU

Cooking Time: 20 minutes

---

3. Quinoa and Vegetable Stuffed Peppers

Ingredients:

- 4 bell peppers, halved and seeds removed
- 1 cup cooked quinoa
- 1 cup cherry tomatoes, diced
- 1/2 cup crumbled feta cheese
- 1/4 cup black olives, sliced
- 2 tablespoons fresh basil, chopped
- 1 tablespoon olive oil
- Salt and pepper to taste

Instructions:

1. Preheat oven to 375°F (190°C).

2. In a bowl, combine cooked quinoa, cherry tomatoes, feta cheese, black olives, fresh basil, olive oil, salt, and pepper.

3. Stuff the halved peppers with the quinoa mixture.

4. Bake for 25-30 minutes or until peppers are tender.

5. Serve warm.

Nutritional Value (per serving):

- Calories: 280

- Protein: 10g

- Fiber: 8g

- Calcium: 120mg

- Vitamin D: 2 IU

Cooking Time: 35 minutes

4. Mediterranean Lentil Soup

Ingredients:

- 1 cup dried green lentils, rinsed
- 1 onion, diced
- 2 carrots, diced
- 2 celery stalks, diced
- 3 cloves garlic, minced
- 1 can (14 oz) diced tomatoes
- 4 cups vegetable broth
- 1 teaspoon ground cumin
- 1 teaspoon ground coriander
- 1/2 teaspoon smoked paprika
- Salt and pepper to taste
- Fresh parsley for garnish

Instructions:

1. In a large pot, sauté onion, carrots, celery, and garlic until softened.

2. Add lentils, diced tomatoes, vegetable broth, cumin, coriander, smoked paprika, salt, and pepper.

3. Bring to a boil, then reduce heat and simmer for 25-30 minutes.

4. Garnish with fresh parsley and Serve hot.

Nutritional Value (per serving): Calories: 240, Protein: 15g, Fiber: 12g, Calcium: 60mg, Vitamin D: 1 IU

Cooking Time: 40 minutes

---

5. Mediterranean Tuna and White Bean Salad

Ingredients:

- 1 can (15 oz) white beans, drained and rinsed
- 1 can (5 oz) tuna, drained
- 1/2 red onion, finely chopped
- 1/4 cup Kalamata olives, sliced
- 1/4 cup cherry tomatoes, halved
- 2 tablespoons extra virgin olive oil
- 1 tablespoon red wine vinegar

- 1 teaspoon dried oregano

- Salt and pepper to taste

Instructions:

1. In a large bowl, combine white beans, tuna, red onion, Kalamata olives, and cherry tomatoes.

2. In a small bowl, whisk together olive oil, red wine vinegar, dried oregano, salt, and pepper.

3. Pour the dressing over the salad and toss to combine.

4. Serve chilled.

Nutritional Value (per serving): Calories: 320, Protein: 20g, Fiber: 9g, Calcium: 80mg, Vitamin D: 1 IU

Cooking Time: 10 minutes

6. Mediterranean Quinoa Salad with Feta and Spinach

Ingredients:

- 1 cup cooked quinoa
- 1 cup fresh spinach, chopped
- 1/2 cup cherry tomatoes, halved
- 1/4 cup crumbled feta cheese
- 2 tablespoons black olives, sliced
- 1 tablespoon extra-virgin olive oil
- 1 tablespoon balsamic vinegar
- Salt and pepper to taste

Instructions:

1. In a bowl, combine cooked quinoa, fresh spinach, cherry tomatoes, feta cheese, and black olives.

2. In a small bowl, whisk together olive oil, balsamic vinegar, salt, and pepper.

3. Pour the dressing over the salad and toss to combine.

4. Serve at room temperature.

Nutritional Value (per serving): Calories: 270, Protein: 8g, Fiber: 6g, Calcium: 120mg, Vitamin D: 2 IU

Cooking Time: 15 minutes

---

7. Mediterranean Eggplant and Chickpea Bake

Ingredients:

- 1 large eggplant, sliced
- 1 can (15 oz) chickpeas, drained and rinsed
- 1 cup cherry tomatoes, halved
- 1/4 cup feta cheese, crumbled
- 2 tablespoons fresh basil, chopped
- 2 tablespoons extra virgin olive oil
- 1 teaspoon dried oregano
- Salt and pepper to taste

Instructions:

1. Preheat oven to 400°F (200°C).

2. Arrange eggplant slices in a baking dish.

3. In a bowl, combine chickpeas, cherry tomatoes, feta cheese, fresh basil, olive oil, dried oregano, salt, and pepper.

4. Spoon the mixture over the eggplant slices.

5. Bake for 25-30 minutes or until eggplant is tender.

6. Serve hot.

Nutritional Value (per serving): Calories: 280, Protein: 12g, Fiber: 10g, Calcium: 120mg, Vitamin D: 2 IU

Cooking Time: 35 minutes

8. Mediterranean Shrimp and Vegetable Skillet

Ingredients:

- 1 lb shrimp, peeled and deveined

- 1 cup cherry tomatoes, halved

- 1 zucchini, sliced

- 1 bell pepper, sliced

- 3 cloves garlic, minced

- 2 tablespoons extra virgin olive oil
- 1 teaspoon dried oregano
- 1/2 teaspoon smoked paprika
- Salt and pepper to taste
- Fresh parsley for garnish

Instructions:

1. In a skillet, heat olive oil over medium heat.
2. Add shrimp and cook until pink, about 2-3 minutes per side.
3. Add cherry tomatoes, zucchini, bell pepper, and minced garlic.
4. Sprinkle with dried oregano, smoked paprika, salt, and pepper.
5. Sauté until vegetables are tender.
6. Garnish with fresh parsley and Serve hot.

Nutritional Value (per serving): Calories: 280, Protein: 25g, Fiber: 6g, Calcium: 80mg, Vitamin D: 2 IU

Cooking Time: 20 minutes

9. Mediterranean Stuffed Portobello Mushrooms

Ingredients:

- 4 large Portobello mushrooms, cleaned and stems removed
- 1 cup quinoa, cooked
- 1/2 cup feta cheese, crumbled
- 1/4 cup black olives, sliced
- 1/4 cup sun-dried tomatoes, chopped
- 2 tablespoons fresh basil, chopped
- 1 tablespoon extra-virgin olive oil
- Salt and pepper to taste

Instructions:

1. Preheat oven to 375°F (190°C).
2. In a bowl, mix cooked quinoa, feta cheese, black olives, sun-dried tomatoes, fresh basil, olive oil, salt, and pepper.
3. Stuff Portobello mushrooms with the quinoa mixture.

4. Bake for 20-25 minutes or until mushrooms are tender.

5. Serve warm.

Nutritional Value (per serving): Calories: 300, Protein: 12g, Fiber: 8g, Calcium: 120mg, Vitamin D: 2 IU

Cooking Time: 30 minutes

---

10. Mediterranean Turkey and Vegetable Skewers

Ingredients:

- 1 lb turkey breast, cut into chunks
- 1 zucchini, sliced
- 1 red onion, cut into wedges
- 1 pint cherry tomatoes
- 2 tablespoons extra virgin olive oil
- 1 teaspoon dried thyme
- 1 teaspoon ground cumin
- Salt and pepper to taste

- Lemon wedges for serving

Instructions:

1. In a bowl, toss turkey, zucchini, red onion, and cherry tomatoes with olive oil, dried thyme, ground cumin, salt, and pepper.

2. Thread onto skewers.

3. Grill skewers over medium heat until turkey is cooked through, about 12-15 minutes.

4. Serve with lemon wedges.

Nutritional Value (per serving): Calories: 260, Protein: 30g, Fiber: 5g, Calcium: 40mg, Vitamin D: 2 IU

Cooking Time: 20 minutes

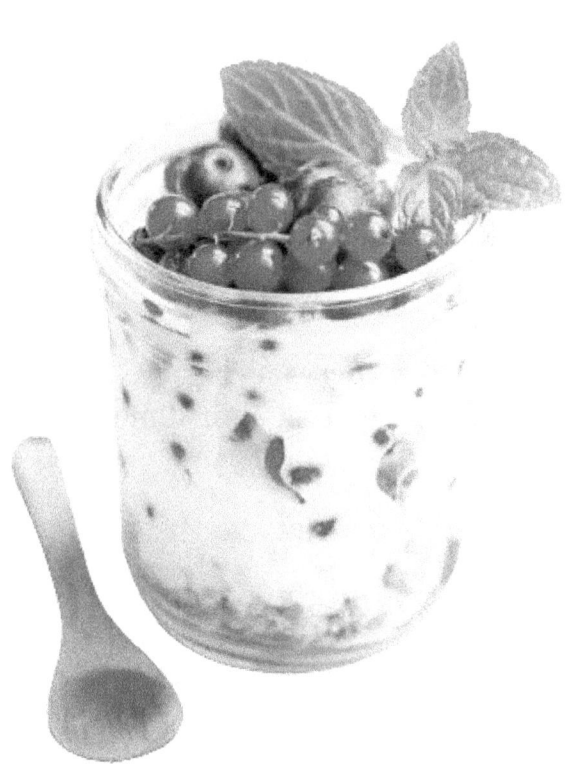

CHAPTER 5: DINNER RECIPES

1. Mediterranean Baked Salmon with Lemon and Dill

Ingredients:

- 4 salmon fillets
- 2 tablespoons extra virgin olive oil
- 1 lemon, sliced
- 2 tablespoons fresh dill, chopped
- Salt and pepper to taste

Instructions:

1. Preheat oven to 400°F (200°C).
2. Place salmon fillets on a baking sheet.
3. Drizzle with olive oil and season with salt and pepper.
4. Top with lemon slices and chopped dill.
5. Bake for 15-18 minutes or until salmon is cooked through.
6. Serve hot.

Nutritional Value (per serving):

- Calories: 300
- Protein: 30g
- Fiber: 2g
- Calcium: 100mg
- Vitamin D: 5 IU

Cooking Time: 20 minutes

2. Mediterranean Quinoa-Stuffed Peppers

Ingredients:

- 4 bell peppers, halved and seeds removed
- 1 cup cooked quinoa
- 1 can (15 oz) chickpeas, drained and rinsed
- 1/2 cup feta cheese, crumbled
- 1/4 cup Kalamata olives, sliced
- 2 tablespoons fresh parsley, chopped
- 2 tablespoons extra virgin olive oil
- Salt and pepper to taste

Instructions:

1. Preheat oven to 375°F (190°C).

2. In a bowl, combine cooked quinoa, chickpeas, feta cheese, Kalamata olives, parsley, olive oil, salt, and pepper.

3. Stuff the halved peppers with the quinoa mixture.

4. Bake for 25-30 minutes or until peppers are tender.

5. Serve warm.

Nutritional Value (per serving):

- Calories: 320

- Protein: 15g

- Fiber: 8g

- Calcium: 120mg

- Vitamin D: 2 IU

Cooking Time: 35 minutes

3. Mediterranean Zucchini Noodles with Pesto and Cherry Tomatoes

Ingredients:

- 4 medium zucchini, spiralized
- 1 cup cherry tomatoes, halved
- 1/4 cup pine nuts, toasted
- 1/2 cup fresh basil leaves
- 1/4 cup Parmesan cheese, grated
- 1 clove garlic
- 1/3 cup extra virgin olive oil
- Salt and pepper to taste

Instructions:

1. In a blender, combine fresh basil, pine nuts, Parmesan cheese, and garlic.
2. While blending, slowly add olive oil until smooth.
3. In a pan, sauté zucchini noodles until tender.
4. Toss with cherry tomatoes and pesto.
5. Season with salt and pepper.

6. Serve immediately.

Nutritional Value (per serving): Calories: 280, Protein: 8g, Fiber: 6g, Calcium: 120mg, Vitamin D: 2 IU

Cooking Time: 15 minutes

---

4. Mediterranean Stuffed Chicken Breast with Spinach and Feta

Ingredients:

- 4 boneless, skinless chicken breasts
- 2 cups fresh spinach, chopped
- 1/2 cup feta cheese, crumbled
- 1 clove garlic, minced
- 1 tablespoon extra-virgin olive oil
- 1 teaspoon dried oregano
- Salt and pepper to taste

Instructions:

1. Preheat oven to 375°F (190°C).

2. In a pan, sauté spinach and garlic in olive oil until wilted.

3. Butterfly chicken breasts and stuff with sautéed spinach and crumbled feta.

4. Season with dried oregano, salt, and pepper.

5. Bake for 25-30 minutes or until chicken is cooked through.

6. Serve hot.

Nutritional Value (per serving):

- Calories: 320

- Protein: 40g

- Fiber: 3g

- Calcium: 120mg

- Vitamin D: 2 IU

Cooking Time: 35 minutes

5. Mediterranean Eggplant and Chickpea Tagine

Ingredients:

- 1 large eggplant, cubed
- 1 can (15 oz) chickpeas, drained and rinsed
- 1 onion, diced
- 2 cloves garlic, minced
- 1 can (14 oz) diced tomatoes
- 1/4 cup raisins
- 2 teaspoons ground cumin
- 1 teaspoon ground coriander
- 1 teaspoon smoked paprika
- 1/2 cup vegetable broth
- 2 tablespoons fresh cilantro, chopped
- 2 tablespoons extra virgin olive oil
- Salt and pepper to taste

Instructions:

1. In a tagine or large pot, sauté onion and garlic in olive oil until softened.

2. Add cubed eggplant, chickpeas, diced tomatoes, raisins, cumin, coriander, smoked paprika, vegetable broth, salt, and pepper.

3. Simmer for 20-25 minutes until eggplant is tender.

4. Garnish with fresh cilantro.

5. Serve hot.

Nutritional Value (per serving):

- Calories: 280

- Protein: 10g

- Fiber: 10g

- Calcium: 120mg

- Vitamin D: 2 IU

Cooking Time: 30 minutes

6. Mediterranean Shrimp and Avocado Salad

Ingredients:

- 1 lb shrimp, peeled and deveined
- 2 avocados, diced
- 1 cup cherry tomatoes, halved
- 1/4 cup red onion, finely chopped
- 2 tablespoons fresh cilantro, chopped
- 2 tablespoons extra virgin olive oil
- 1 tablespoon red wine vinegar
- Salt and pepper to taste

Instructions:

1. In a pan, cook shrimp until pink, about 2-3 minutes per side.

2. In a large bowl, combine shrimp, diced avocados, cherry tomatoes, red onion, and cilantro.

3. In a small bowl, whisk together olive oil, red wine vinegar, salt, and pepper.

4. Pour the dressing over the salad and toss to combine.

5. Serve chilled.

Nutritional Value (per serving):

- Calories: 300

- Protein: 25g

- Fiber: 8g

- Calcium: 60mg

- Vitamin D: 2 IU

Cooking Time: 15 minutes

Ingredients:

- 4 cod fillets
- 1 cup cherry tomatoes, diced
- 1/2 cucumber, diced
- 1/4 cup red onion, finely chopped
- 2 tablespoons Kalamata olives, sliced
- 2 tablespoons fresh parsley, chopped
- 2 tablespoons extra virgin olive oil
- 1 tablespoon red wine vinegar
- Salt and pepper to taste

Instructions:

1. Preheat oven to 400°F (200°C).

2. Season cod fillets with salt and pepper.

3. Place cod on a baking sheet and bake for 15-18 minutes or until cooked through.

4. In a bowl, combine diced cherry tomatoes, cucumber, red onion, Kalamata olives, parsley, olive oil, red wine vinegar, salt, and pepper to make the salsa.

5. Top baked cod with Mediterranean salsa.

6. Serve hot.

Nutritional Value (per serving):

- Calories: 280
- Protein: 30g
- Fiber: 5g
- Calcium: 60mg
- Vitamin D: 3 IU
- Cooking Time: 20 minutes

Ingredients:

- 1 cup cooked lentils
- 1 zucchini, sliced
- 1 bell pepper, sliced
- 1 cup cherry tomatoes, halved
- 1/4 cup feta cheese, crumbled
- 2 tablespoons fresh oregano, chopped
- 2 tablespoons extra virgin olive oil
- 1 tablespoon balsamic vinegar
- Salt and pepper to taste

Instructions:

1. In a pan, sauté zucchini, bell pepper, and cherry tomatoes in olive oil until tender.

2. Add cooked lentils and stir-fry until heated through.

3. Drizzle with balsamic vinegar and season with salt and pepper.

4. Top with crumbled feta cheese and fresh oregano.

5. Serve warm.

Nutritional Value (per serving): Calories: 320, Protein: 15g, Fiber: 12g, Calcium: 120mg, Vitamin D: 2 IU

Cooking Time: 15 minutes

---

9. Mediterranean Turkey and Vegetable Meatballs

Ingredients:

- 1 lb ground turkey
- 1 zucchini, grated
- 1 carrot, grated
- 1/4 cup breadcrumbs
- 2 cloves garlic, minced
- 2 tablespoons fresh mint, chopped
- 1 tablespoon extra-virgin olive oil

- 1 teaspoon ground cumin
- 1/2 teaspoon smoked paprika
- Salt and pepper to taste

Instructions:

1. Preheat oven to 375°F (190°C).

2. In a bowl, combine ground turkey, grated zucchini, grated carrot, breadcrumbs, minced garlic, chopped mint, olive oil, cumin, smoked paprika, salt, and pepper.

3. Shape into meatballs and place on a baking sheet.

4. Bake for 20-25 minutes or until cooked through. Serve hot.

Nutritional Value (per serving):

- Calories: 280
- Protein: 25g
- Fiber: 4g
- Calcium: 60mg
- Vitamin D: 2 IU

Cooking Time: 25 minutes

10. Mediterranean Vegetable and Chickpea Couscous

Ingredients:

- 1 cup whole wheat couscous, cooked
- 1 can (15 oz) chickpeas, drained and rinsed
- 1 zucchini, diced
- 1 red bell pepper, diced
- 1 cup cherry tomatoes, halved
- 2 tablespoons fresh parsley, chopped
- 2 tablespoons extra virgin olive oil
- 1 tablespoon lemon juice
- 1 teaspoon ground cumin
- Salt and pepper to taste

Instructions:

1. In a bowl, combine cooked couscous, chickpeas, diced zucchini, diced red bell pepper, cherry tomatoes, parsley, olive oil, lemon juice, cumin, salt, and pepper.

2. Toss to combine.

3. Serve at room temperature.

Nutritional Value (per serving):

- Calories: 300

- Protein: 12g

- Fiber: 10g

- Calcium: 80mg

- Vitamin D: 2 IU

Cooking Time: 15 minutes

These dinner recipes are not only delicious but also rich in nutrients that can be beneficial for individuals managing Rheumatoid Arthritis. As always, consult with a healthcare professional or a registered dietitian to ensure these recipes align with individual health needs and dietary restrictions.

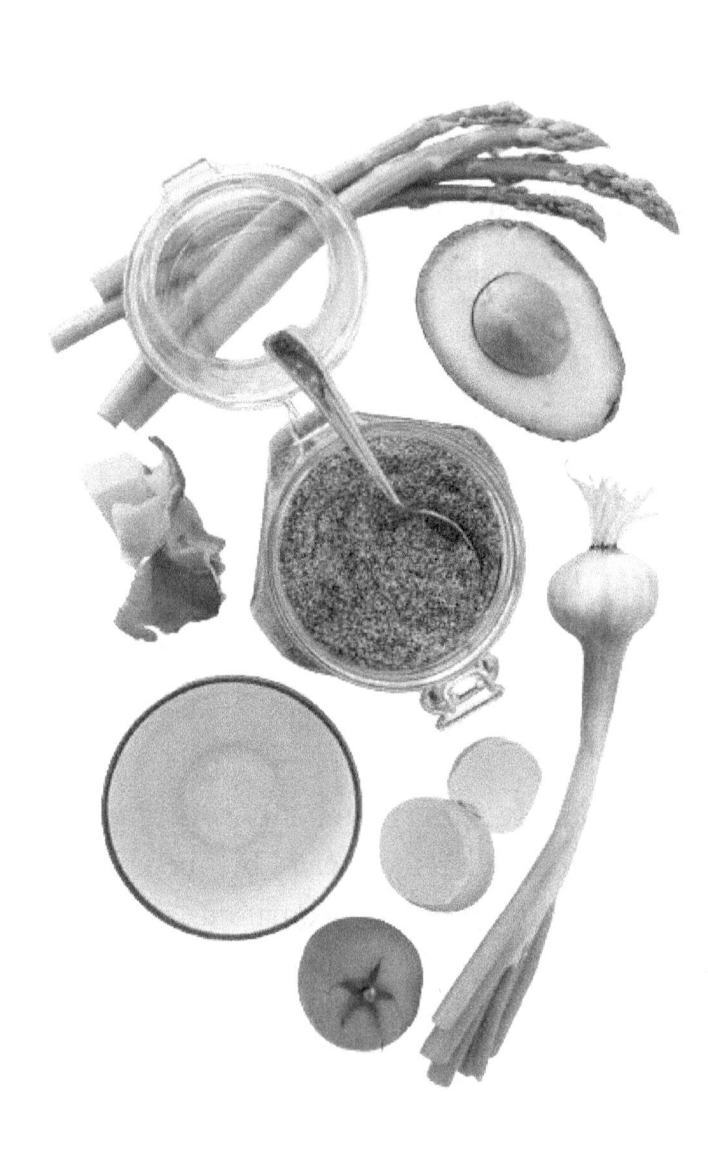

CONCLUSION

In conclusion, the "Mediterranean Diet Cookbook for Rheumatoid Arthritis" serves not only as a culinary guide but as a beacon of hope for those seeking natural remedies to manage and combat the challenges posed by Rheumatoid Arthritis. Through carefully crafted recipes, we've explored the vibrant and flavorful world of Mediterranean cuisine, handpicking ingredients rich in anti-inflammatory properties, calcium, and vitamin D to enhance bone health.

As a nutritionist with a profound commitment to the well-being of individuals, I've witnessed the transformative power of this diet firsthand. The journey recounted, particularly the triumph over Rheumatoid Arthritis by my sister Linda, stands as a testament to the potential benefits of embracing a diet rooted in the Mediterranean tradition. From breakfast to dinner, each recipe is meticulously designed not only to tantalize taste buds but also to nourish the body, promoting overall health and mitigating the impact of this challenging condition.

As you embark on this culinary journey, envision a life where your meals become a source of healing, resilience, and joy. Embrace the simplicity and richness of Mediterranean flavors, savoring the diverse textures and aromas that accompany each dish. Remember, adopting a Mediterranean diet is not just a change in your daily meals; it's an investment in your well-being. Let this cookbook be your companion in the kitchen, guiding you towards a lifestyle that not only manages Rheumatoid Arthritis but elevates your entire sense of health and vitality.

In your hands, you hold not just a cookbook but a pathway to a healthier, more vibrant future. May the recipes within these pages be the first step on your journey to better well-being. Here's to a life filled with delicious, nutritious, and inflammation-fighting meals.

Bon appétit and a healthier, happier you!

MEAL PLANNER

DATE:

	BREAKFAST	LUNCH	DINNER	SHOPPING LIST
MON				
TUES				
WED				
THURS				
FRI				
SAT				
SUN				

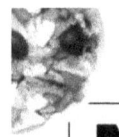

MEAL PLANNER

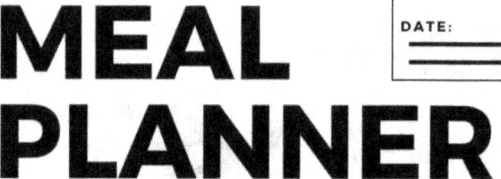

	BREAKFAST	LUNCH	DINNER	SHOPPING LIST
MON				
TUES				
WED				
THURS				
FRI				
SAT				
SUN				

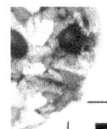

MEAL
PLANNER

DATE: _____

	BREAKFAST	LUNCH	DINNER	SHOPPING LIST
MON				
TUES				
WED				
THURS				
FRI				
SAT				
SUN				

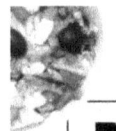

MEAL
PLANNER

DATE: _____

	BREAKFAST	LUNCH	DINNER	SHOPPING LIST
MON				
TUES				
WED				
THURS				
FRI				
SAT				
SUN				

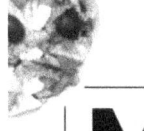

MEAL
PLANNER

DATE: _____

	BREAKFAST	LUNCH	DINNER	SHOPPING LIST
MON				
TUES				
WED				
THURS				
FRI				
SAT				
SUN				

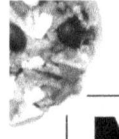

MEAL
PLANNER

DATE: _____

	BREAKFAST	LUNCH	DINNER	SHOPPING LIST
MON				
TUES				
WED				
THURS				
FRI				
SAT				
SUN				

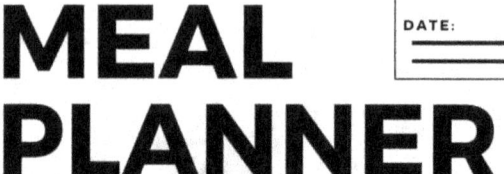

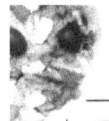

MEAL
PLANNER

DATE:

	BREAKFAST	LUNCH	DINNER	SHOPPING LIST
MON				
TUES				
WED				
THURS				
FRI				
SAT				
SUN				

MEAL
PLANNER

DATE: _____

	BREAKFAST	LUNCH	DINNER	SHOPPING LIST
MON				
TUES				
WED				
THURS				
FRI				
SAT				
SUN				

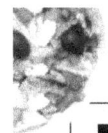

MEAL
PLANNER

DATE: _____

	BREAKFAST	LUNCH	DINNER	SHOPPING LIST
MON				
TUES				
WED				
THURS				
FRI				
SAT				
SUN				

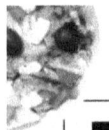

MEAL
PLANNER

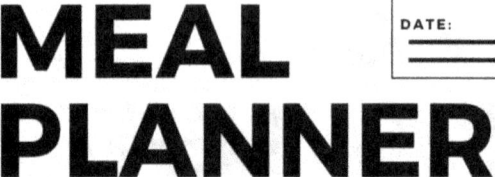

	BREAKFAST	LUNCH	DINNER	SHOPPING LIST
MON				
TUES				
WED				
THURS				
FRI				
SAT				
SUN				

MEAL
PLANNER

DATE:

	BREAKFAST	LUNCH	DINNER	SHOPPING LIST
MON				
TUES				
WED				
THURS				
FRI				
SAT				
SUN				

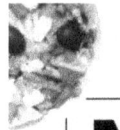

MEAL
PLANNER

DATE:

	BREAKFAST	LUNCH	DINNER	SHOPPING LIST
MON				
TUES				
WED				
THURS				
FRI				
SAT				
SUN				

www.ingramcontent.com/pod-product-compliance
Lightning Source LLC
Chambersburg PA
CBHW071101290526
45795CB00004B/1611